Ultimate Anti-Aging
*S*ECRETS

Everything You Need to Know
to Maintain Youth at Any Age

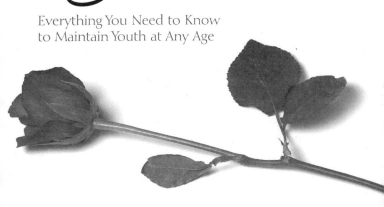

PETER LAMAS

Strength
& Honor

BRONZE
BOW PUB.

The information in this book is for educational purposes only and is not recommended as a means of diagnosing or treating an illness. Neither the publisher nor author is engaged in rendering professional advice or services to the individual reader. All matters regarding physical and mental health should be supervised by a health practitioner knowledgeable in treating that particular condition. Neither the author nor the publisher shall be liable or responsible for any loss, injury, or damage allegedly arising from any information or suggestion in this book.

Ultimate Anti-Aging Secrets
Copyright © 2003 Peter Lamas
All Scripture quotations, unless otherwise indicated, are taken from the *Holy Bible, New International Version®*. NIV®.
Copyright © 1973, 1978, 1984 by International Bible Society.
Used by permission of Zondervan Publishing House. All rights reserved.
ISBN 1-932458-05-0
Published by Bronze Bow Publishing, Inc.,
2600 East 26th Street, Minneapolis, MN 55406.
You can reach us on the Internet at
WWW.BRONZEBOWPUBLISHING.COM
Literary development and cover/interior design by Koechel Peterson & Associates, Inc., Minneapolis, Minnesota.
Manufactured in the United States of America

CONTENTS

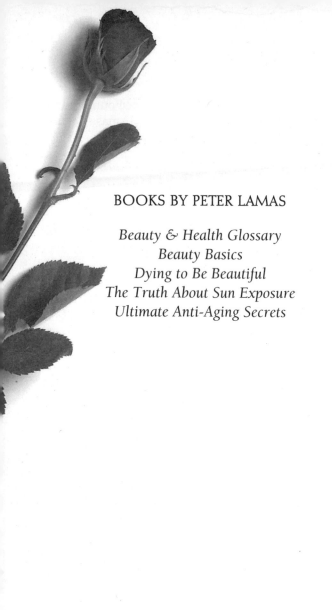

BOOKS BY PETER LAMAS

Beauty & Health Glossary
Beauty Basics
Dying to Be Beautiful
The Truth About Sun Exposure
Ultimate Anti-Aging Secrets

ABOUT THE AUTHOR

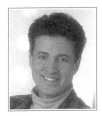

PETER LAMAS is Founder and Chairman of Lamas Beauty International, one of the fastest growing and respected natural beauty products manufacturers in the United States. He has been a major force in the beauty industry for more than 30 years. Peter's career began in New York City as an apprentice to trailblazers Vidal Sassoon and Paul Mitchell, providing the opportunity to work with some of the most famous and beautiful women of our time. His expertise in the areas of hair care, skin care, and makeup has given him a client list that reads like a *who's who of celebrities.*

His work has spanned numerous films, television, video, and print projects, including designing the gorgeous makeup used on the set of the epic film, *Titanic.* Peter has worked with the great names in fashion and beauty photography, including Richard Avedon, Irving Penn, and Francesco Scavullo. His work has been seen in photo shoots in leading magazines, such as *Vogue, Harper's Bazaar, Glamour,* and *Mademoiselle.*

Peter regularly appears on television and in the media in North and South America, Europe, and Asia. He travels extensively across the globe, speaking to women of many different cultures about how they can realize their potential to be beautiful both inside and out, especially educating them about the facts and myths on beauty products.

Cuban born Peter Lamas immigrated to New

York in 1961. Several years later, while pursuing a career as a commercial artist, Peter decided to finance his education by doing hair and makeup. As a result, he discovered he not only had a flair for doing hair and makeup, but he truly enjoyed helping each client look her best.

Peter's life has been dedicated to helping women feel good about themselves, by helping them realize their vast potential for personal beauty. To him, beauty is not just about the perfect haircut or makeup; it's about the full package. He can make just about any woman look absolutely stunning; but if she doesn't feel beautiful, she won't be. Beauty is very personal, and contrary to the cliché "that beauty is in the eye of the beholder," he came to realize that it is also in the eye of the possessor, because what makes us truly attractive to others is the projection of our self-esteem. Grace, confidence, and personality play a major role in attractiveness.

Peter's web site, www.lamasbeauty.com, is one of the largest women's beauty and health information resources on the Internet, through which he and a host of contributing writers keep women and men informed on important beauty and health topics.

Mr. Lamas is an innovative product developer in the cosmetics industry and recently received the distinguished honor from *Health Magazine* for developing the "Best Moisturizer of the Year." You can learn more about Peter's company, Lamas Beauty International, by visiting www.lamasbeauty.com or emailing him directly at peterlamas@lamasbeauty.com.

Youthful, Vibrant,
AND HEALTHY

> But those who hope in the Lord will renew
> their strength. They will soar on wings like
> eagles; they will run and not grow weary,
> they will walk and not be faint.
> —Isaiah 40:31

WHEN the Italians lift their glasses at a wedding and toast "cent'anni," it means to 100 years. What was once mostly a wishful toast has now become a reality. With modern advances in science continuing to extend life expectancies, the century mark is very much a possibility. Remarkably, since 1900 we have gained an average of 110 days a year and our life expectancy in the United States increased 62 percent. Experts predict that the number of people who live to celebrate a one hundredth birthday will increase over fifty times in the next 20 years. Healthcare advances, better education, and increased financial and informational resources will enable many of us to live well past 100.

We live in a fascinating time when scientists from several different fields are close to breakthroughs in defying the aging process. Legendary biochemist Bruce Ames has proven that aging occurs in our body through a process characterized by our immune system beginning to break down through free radicals. Genetic material in our body's 100 trillion cells gets damaged, which not only decreases our energy levels but eventually can lead to cell mutation (which can cause cancer) and cell death. Ames is confident that research will yield nutrients that not only repair that damage but renew those cells.

Meanwhile, molecular biologist Judith Campisi is researching how to keep cells from aging. Breakthrough advances in cellular research since 1990 has shown that we age because our cells stop dividing over time and start to malfunction, not because the cells die. Campisi is looking for a way to alter genes to extend the life span.

Still others are pursuing research on DHEA, which is an adrenal hormone naturally produced in large quantities in our youth that declines around the age of 25. And then there is all sorts of research that surrounds hGH (Human Growth Hormone), which also decreases with age (at a rate of approximately 14 percent per decade). I am concerned about the long-term effects for those who are taking hGH and DHEA supplements today as some research has shown potential damage related to it.

And while these various research projects may lead to the day of extended longevity, and perhaps the day is soon coming when we will be able to replace worn-out parts of our body, what is most important today is that as we age we continue to be youthful, vibrant, and healthy for all of those added years. We have the power to do something about adding quality to our years. Through the wealth of studies that have been done on the secrets to anti-aging, we can assess the daily changes we can make in our lives to maintain our youth at any age.

CHAPTER ONE

Anti-Aging Begins
WITH ATTITUDE

Hippocrates, the Father of Medicine, knew about anti-aging somewhere around 400 B.C., so I'm not breaking new ground when I say that anti-aging begins with attitude. Hippocrates noted that certain individuals were more susceptible to illness, and that personality type and attitude were the keys. It's a well corroborated fact that if you approach life and its stresses with a positive attitude that refuses to give in to the pressures, that attitude will have a marked affect on the health of your body, which in turn slows the aging process.

"By thinking optimistically," says Karen Asp, noted health and fitness writer and lamasbeauty.com contributing writer, "you can increase your odds of living longer. A recent study at the Mayo Clinic found that pessimism is a risk factor for premature death, even when other risk factors such as age and sex are discarded. If you're more optimistic, start seeing the glass as half full rather than half empty, you'll handle stress better, get sick less often, and experience success in work, school, sports, relationships with your family and friends, and everything else you do." That's a formula that rolls back the aging process.

CHOOSING OPTIMISM

King Solomon made this classic statement about man: "For as he thinks in his heart, so is he" (Proverbs 23:7). The attitude you bring to daily life is a choice you make. You choose to be positive and happy, and you choose to be the opposite. But to be negative leads to long, tough days that sap your whole well-being. Life is full of problems and bad days, which a bad attitude only makes worse. Some days are overwhelming, and how you deal with them makes all the difference.

It is our nature to want to enjoy a long and happy life. But many of us seek to find that happiness in all manner of destructive ways. We try to find satisfaction in a job, or in a person, or in a house, or in a position, or in a bottle or a pill, only to be utterly disappointed. Rather than grasping for something to fulfill us from the outside, we are constantly brought back to the fact that joy and peace and fulfillment must come from within. The choice is ours. Here are some ways you can do that:

- Feed your mind with the truth and positive thoughts. A great place to look is the Bible, which says, "Whatever is true, whatever is noble, whatever is right, whatever is pure, whatever is lovely, whatever is admirable—if anything is excellent or praiseworthy—think about such things" (Philippians 4:8). Conversely, it will keep dark and negative thoughts away.

- Live every day on the basis that it's a gift you've been given. There's a beautiful little gift book from Hallmark called *If Only I Knew* by Lance Wubbels that speaks to this in a profound manner. Because everything in life can change in a heartbeat, we must make the most of the moments God gives us.

- Accept the fact that there will be difficult days and that no one is emotionally up all the time. It is foolish to expect everything to work out the way we want or to think we will not be deeply challenged to persevere and pass through problems.

- Pay attention to your personal needs. If you take care of yourself first, you'll have plenty of enthusiasm, energy, and optimism to give to others.
- Celebrate the power of choice. My parents gave up almost everything to came to America rather than be oppressed in Cuba under Castro. Don't play the victim. If something in your life needs a change, take action and go for it. Listen to your dreams and go after them.

Here are some more ways to make your world brighter from Karen Asp:

- Find positive friends. If you want to soar with eagles, you have to stop hanging out with the ducks.
- Let go of things that drain your energy, such as worry.
- Enjoy the simple things. There's a cap to how much happiness fancy cars and big homes will give you. But there's no limit to the joy you'll get from playing with your kids, watching hummingbirds flutter at the feeder, or gazing at fluffy clouds.
- The more you laugh the better you'll feel. When

you laugh, endorphins, the "feel good" hormones, rush through your body like a burst of happy energy.

- Get moving. Remember those endorphins? You'll feel them when you exercise, whether you're walking the dog or raking leaves.
- Indulge your best passions. Enjoy what you love to do and don't feel guilty about doing it.
- Take the challenge. Put such an emphasis on the positive that you're ready to tackle anything.

CHAPTER TWO

The Power of a
NUTRITIOUS DIET

HUNDREDS of health studies confirm the power of a nutritious diet in the battle against aging by preventing disease from ever starting in our body. A balanced diet is the foundation of good health and anti-aging. What you choose to eat has the power to lower or raise the risk of heart disease, cancer, obesity, hormonal imbalances, diabetes, and other chronic diseases. It is estimated that 30 to 40 percent of all cancers are related to diet. With over 16 million Americans now being affected by diabetes and an estimated

300,000 Americans dying prematurely each year of diseases caused by being very overweight, nutrition is the key.

Evelyn Gavalas is the author of *Secrets of Fat-Free Greek Cooking* and has written several diet and food articles for my web site, lamasbeauty.com. I highly recommend that you visit the site and read her insight. I agree with her when she writes: "A number of health and longevity studies show the vegetarian, Mediterranean, and Asian eating styles to be the world's healthiest diets, increasing life expectancy and lowering the risk of many of the diseases that afflict Americans. These diets are low in saturated fat and high in plant-based foods that are rich in cancer-preventing phytochemicals, immune-boosting antioxidants, and colon-cleansing fiber.... Vitamin- and antioxidant-rich fresh fruit and/or vegetables should be eaten at every meal, with daily servings of fresh fish (which supplies beneficial omega-3 fatty acids), high fiber grains and beans, soy foods, and limited dairy and sweets. Daily servings of low-glycemic index, complex carbohydrate rich foods lower the incidence of diabetes, insulin resistance, and heart disease, as well as encourage weight loss and maintenance."

WHICH DIET IS BEST?

With myriads upon myriads of diets available, and having watched myriads of clients chase one diet after another, my perspective is that you should establish a balanced diet that works for you and that you hold to it consistently. I have seen too many fad weight-loss programs that usually push one food group to the extreme (especially protein), which in fact forced my clients to burn up muscle tissue which was later replaced by fat and left behind dreaded lines, wrinkles, and loose skin. The secret is rather to provide your body with the right building materials in the right portions.

I advise clients to consider everything they eat. I ask them to always pause and think about what that specific food will do for and to them, and to eat accordingly. It's amazing what happens when you do that. And I believe that portion control is a major factor that will help you reach and maintain your ideal weight. It's important to eat smaller portions of more kinds of plant-based, nutritious foods. Portion control is easy when you include whole foods, herbs, and seasonings high in flavor and variety, so you can enjoy your meals and never feel deprived without sacrificing valuable nutrients.

A BALANCED DIET

Most health and nutrition experts agree that a daily balanced diet should contain the following:

- **2 to 3 servings of lean protein.** The body requires protein, especially to build muscle, but only needs a modest amount (55 grams). Additional protein is stored in fat. Instead of red meat, opt for skinless organic chicken or turkey or fish. Eggs, beans, and tofu are also good sources.

- **2 to 3 servings of low-fat dairy products.** These are rich in minerals and some fat-soluble vitamins, but we usually overindulge. Look for skim milk, low- or no-fat yogurt, cottage cheese, and goat's cheese. I recommend organic cow's milk and dairy if you can get it. Non-organic contains growth hormones, medications, antibiotics, and pesticides at low levels that can affect your health.

- **3 to 5 servings of vegetables.** They are full of vitamins and minerals, low on calories, and at the same time filling. Try to eat fresh or frozen to maximize their food values and internal cleansing action. Consider sea vegetables, which are rich sources of vitamins, minerals, phytochemicals, and protein. Studies suggest sea vegetables in the diet may be why the incidence of breast and colon cancer is lower among Japanese people.

Space does not permit describing all the benefits you receive from vegetables.

- **2 to 4 servings of fruit.** Fuel your body with incredibly high amounts of vitamins, minerals, and enzymes that also help you lose weight while adding muscle mass. Fruit is nature's delicious fast food.
- **6 to 12 servings of whole-grain breads, grains, pastas, rice, or cereals.** Stick with these slow burning, complex carbohydrates to sustain your body and mind with energy. They are a good source of antioxidants and phytoestrogens and promote healthy elimination, good memory, clear thinking, and quick reflexes.

If you stick within the framework of these time-tested guidelines, you'll be amazed at the results. Within these categories are a host of delicious foods that provide your body with everything you need for health and vitality, and because you love the food, you will stay with the system. Keep it simple, and keep it delightfully delicious.

STAY AWAY FROM SUGAR AND PROCESSED FOODS

To be healthy, keep your intake of bad simple carbohydrates (sugars) as low as possible. When you consume a substantial amount of sugar, a heavy dose of glucose gets released into your bloodstream, which causes your body to produce high levels of insulin. This, in turn, inhibits hormone-sensitive lipase, the enzyme that is responsible for draining fat from the cells. Which is the opposite of what you want.

Stay away from processed foods as much as possible. They may contain hidden ingredients labeled as "natural flavoring" that are chemicals. If possible, stay away from white breads, white pasta, or white rice—they have been processed and refined into starches that behave as sugars.

EATING TIPS

- Never skip breakfast. Make it a power meal with high quality foods that fuel your body and brain.
- Eat small meals, more often, if possible—5 to 6 times a day. Don't go more than 4 hours without eating something.
- The later you eat in the evening, the less likely you are of burning up those calories. If you can eat by 6 p.m., do it.
- Go for foods rich in color.
- Always avoid fast food and junk food—period.
- Drink lots of green tea. It has heart and cancer-

protecting properties and contains polyphenols, important antioxidants that have been shown to lower cholesterol, prevent cancer, and improve fat metabolism.

- Eat lots of beans. They are loaded with nutrients and help lower cholesterol and blood sugar as well as prevent cancer. Be creative and use them in pastas, salads, soups, stews, and dips.

- Give soy a try. It lowers the risk of heart disease, cancers, and digestive disorders, eases the symptoms of menopause and PMS, and guards against osteoporosis. Fortified soy milk is a healthy substitute for cow's milk, while tofu and textured soy protein (TSP) deliver high-quality protein in place of meat.

- Your body requires up to 30 percent of healthy fat into your diet. Healthy fats contain omega-3 and omega-9 fatty acids, which have been shown to prevent heart attacks, obesity, diabetes, depression, breast and prostate cancer. Olive and flaxseed oils and seeds and nuts are good sources. Many varieties of fish are low in fat and cholesterol and contain a high concentration of healthful omega-3 fatty acids (salmon, halibut, mackerel, sardines, and tuna). Fish is also a rich source of protein and provides 100 percent of daily Vitamin D and the antioxidant mineral selenium (which aids in preventing hair and nail loss) and 25 percent of daily Vitamin B.

To live long and be happier and healthier, make wise food choices that will benefit your entire life. Instead of a beef taco, go for a bean burrito. By choosing a veggie burger, spinach salad, and a fruit smoothie instead of a cheeseburger, French fries, and a milkshake, you're making an important choice that saves the body . . . and maybe even saves your life.

CHAPTER THREE

Exercise — the Silver Bullet of ANTI-AGING

As important as a healthy diet is, if there is one silver bullet for anti-aging, it is consistent exercise. Without exercise, even the best of diets is like a race car without an engine—it goes nowhere. Every benefit of exercise takes a significant bite out of the aging process:

- Reduces your risk for developing heart disease (the leading killer in the U.S.), stroke, bad cholesterol (LDL), diabetes, high blood pressure, colon cancer, and breast cancer. How's that for a healthy starter?

- Reduces your stress by activating your endorphins, causing a natural high and a sense of well-being, which also improves your circulation, digestion, and mental processes. Reduces your symptoms of depression and anxiety.
- Helps develop lean muscle, reduce body fat, build and maintain healthy bones, muscles, and joints, and delay the development of osteoporosis.
- Strengthens your immune system to fight illness and stress and increases the detoxification rate as well as the cellular turnover rate.
- Reduces your appetite while increasing your sex drive. That's a nice trade.
- Helps normalize women's hormone levels, reducing problems with PMS and menopause.

Despite these amazing benefits, sedentary Americans remain stuck on the couch. One out every three people you meet is overweight, two out of five will die of heart disease, six out of ten will resort to medication to feel better, and 14 percent suffer from depression.

SO WHERE DO YOU START?

I am not a proponent of working out in a gym for

hours every day. I am for consistent aerobic exercise. In general, an aerobic exercise is any exercise that can be continued for 20 minutes or longer, uses large muscle groups, and is rhythmic in nature. The most popular aerobic exercises include fast walking, running, cycling, rowing, dance, calisthenics, tennis, basketball, rollerblading, martial arts, and on and on.

If done consistently, and to me it's all about consistency, aerobic exercise trains the heart, lungs, and cardiovascular system to process and deliver the oxygen that burns calories. And when you burn calories, the body must compensate for the extra energy being used, so the mitochondria inside your cells divide. Since the mitochondria act as our power plants, burning fuel, they divide as you exercise, burning twice as much. Nothing else will do that. It's that simple.

If you have not been exercising, consider starting with 3 to 5 aerobic sessions per week for a duration of at least 20 minutes. If you can double that to 40 minutes, it's worth it. I recommend that you use walking as your beginning point. It is a very doable exercise with all the benefits listed previously. If you are obese or weak, I recommend you get John Peterson's workout book, *Pushing Yourself to Power*, that has a chapter designated with special exercises to bring you up to the point where you can enter into an aerobic program. He also has a set of special exercises for super joints and lifelong pain-free mobility that are essential to anti-aging.

Ultimately, the goal is for you to add lean, toned muscle. Muscle is valuable for many reasons, and especially for burning calories. Be encouraged by this: 1 pound of muscle burns about 35 calories per day, while 1 pound of fat burns only 2 calories. If you add 10 pounds of muscle, you'll naturally burn 350 calories more per day, and every 10 days you'll burn off a pound of fat naturally (there are 3,500 calories stored in 1 pound of fat).

So make the choice to start exercising today. Make a lifelong change that will enhance every facet of your life!

CHAPTER FOUR

Vitamins and
MINERALS

VITAMINS and minerals are essential anti-aging fighters, and most of the supply of the essential nutrients your body requires is found in a healthy, balanced diet. But there are many reasons to supplement your diet with vitamins and minerals. Because of the quality of our food, even when we eat the right foods we may not be getting the right nutrients. Most foods are depleted of nutrients, vitamins, and minerals. Because of that we must take extra supplements.

Most of us do not realize that if we are lacking in minerals, very few of the nutrients we ingest will be absorbed, so a liquid mineral supplement is mandatory in most cases. Also, stress alone can deplete all your water-soluble vitamins within one to two hours, particularly B vitamins that provide the body's peace and much more. A B-complex, food-based vitamin is an absolute must.

In her book *How to Feel Great All the Time,* Dr. Valerie Saxion says, "Vitamins are a group of organic compounds that are essential for normal growth, development, and metabolism. They are produced by living material, plants and animals, as compared to minerals that come from the soil. Insufficient supplies of any of the vitamins result in specific deficiency diseases. Vitamins function along with enzymes in chemical reactions necessary for human bodily function, including energy production. Vitamins and enzymes also work together to act as a catalyst in speeding up the making or breaking of chemical bonds that join molecules together.

"Vitamins are classified into two groups. Fat-soluble vitamins (A, D, E, and K) dissolve in fat and are stored in the fatty parts of the liver and other tissues. Water-soluble vitamins (the Bs and C) dissolve in water and are not stored by the body to any great extent.

"Minerals function, along with vitamins, as components of body enzymes. Minerals are needed for proper composition of teeth and bone and blood. They are important to the production of hormones and enzymes and in the creation of antibodies. Some minerals (calcium, potassium, and sodium) have electrical charges that act as a magnet to attract other electrically charged substances to form complex molecules, conduct electrical impulses along nerves, and transport substances in and out of the cells."

Deficiencies of minerals are more prevalent than deficiencies of vitamins. If you are a vegetarian, elderly, on a low-calorie diet, taking certain drugs, or pregnant, you are at an increased risk. Keep in mind that some minerals compete for absorption, so taking a large dose of one mineral may deplete your body's absorption of another mineral.

THE ROLE OF VITAMINS

Susan Kleinman, who writes about health and women's issues and is a lamasbeauty.com correspondent, says, "Vitamins C and E and beta-carotene, which attack free radicals and keep your cells healthier, can extend your youthful life significantly. According to a UCLA study of 11,500 people who took over 500 milligrams a day of Vitamin C and drank 8 ounces of orange juice daily, the men added five years to their lives, on average, and the women added a year, while cutting their risk of stroke and heart attack by 25 percent. In addition to eating a healthy diet with lots of green and orange vegetables, take a multivitamin daily."

Vitamin E is a potent antioxidant that countless research has shown is good for the heart, the brain, and the immune system. Applied topically, it is also an excellent skin moisturizer and an aid in the healing of scars.

Vitamin C is a vital antioxidant and champion of the immune system that helps reduce the risk of cancer and cardiovascular diseases. My *Pro-Vita C Moisturizer SPF 15* won the prestigious *Health Magazine's* "Best Moisturizer of the Year Award." It protects skin during the daytime with a multi-action combination of natural antioxidants that break down free radicals before they can damage skin. A high percentage of highly absorbable Vitamin C invigorates collagen and elastin reproduction, which helps increase firmness, while also helping to decrease hyperpigmentation (especially freckles and age spots).

Carotenoids have been identified as the pigments that give fruits and vegetables their vivid colors. A mixed carotenoid supplement, including beta-carotene (precursor to Vitamin A), lutein and lycopene are powerful antioxidants that boost immune function and help prevent cancer, heart disease, and macular degeneration. Topical Vitamin A, found in skin formulas such as Retin-A and Renova, are powerful treatments for acne and sun-damaged, dry skin.

Vitamin B-6, which is found especially in fish, poultry, whole-grain cereals, most vegetables, meat, and eggs may be a woman's best friend. Recent studies show that B6 may help alleviate premenstrual symptoms such as bloating, irritability, depression, and fatigue.

Space does not allow us to highlight the unlimited anti-aging benefits of the 13 vitamins our bodies require. Every vitamin has a specific function that nothing else can replace. And, if any vitamin is lacking, it can hinder the function of another. Always take a food-based multivitamin capsule that covers all the bases.

THE ROLE OF MINERALS

According to the U.S. Department of Agriculture, the average American consumes only about 60 percent of the essential minerals their bodies need. And without sufficient amounts of minerals, you can't absorb your vitamins! Which is why I'm stressing them here. Here are 10 minerals that Dr. Valerie Saxion says you can't do without in the battle against aging.

Calcium is absolutely vital for strong bones and teeth and for the battle against osteoporosis. It helps the body maintain a regular heartbeat, aids in the transmission of nerve impulses, lowers bad cholesterol, helps prevent cardiovascular disease, and wards off muscle cramps.

Copper aids in the formation of bone, hemoglobin, and red blood cells. It's also involved in the body's healing process and energy production and is required for healthy nerves and joints.

Iodine is so essential for mental and physical development that if children are lacking in it, they can end up mentally challenged. Sufficient iodine is necessary for a healthy thyroid, and in trace amounts, iodine helps to metabolize excess fat.

Magnesium is a vital catalyst in enzyme activity, particularly those involved in the production of energy. It helps the body absorb calcium and potassium and helps prevent muscle weakness and twitching, while maintaining the body's proper pH balance. A deficiency of magnesium interferes with the transmission of nerve and muscle impulses, resulting in irritability and nervousness. If you suffer from PMS or depression, this mineral could be your magic bullet.

Manganese is a must-have for iron. Minute quantities are required for the metabolism of protein and fat, healthy nerves, a healthy immune system, and proper regulation of blood sugar. The body also uses it to produce energy, and it's required for normal bone growth, reproduction, the formation of cartilage, and the production of synovial fluid, which lubricates the body's joints and tendons.

Phosphorus assists the body both in utilizing vitamins and converting food to energy. It's needed for bone and teeth formation and cell growth and helps both heart and kidney function. Deficiencies can lead to anxiety, bone pain, fatigue, irregular breathing, irritability, numbness, skin sensitivity, trembling, and weakness.

Silicon is a mineral superhero! It helps the body absorb calcium and plays a major role in the prevention of cardiovascular disease. Since it counteracts the effects of aluminum, it is essential in the prevention of Alzheimer's disease and osteoporosis. It also stimulates the immune system and inhibits the aging process in tissues.

Sodium assists in regulating the body's water balance and blood pH. It helps maintain normal heart rhythm and is necessary for proper stomach, nerve, and muscle function.

Sulphur is not only necessary for the formation of collagen for bones and connective tissue but promotes healthy nails, skin, and hair. It also disinfects blood, helps the body resist bacteria, and protects the protoplasm of cells. Sulphur slows down the aging process by protecting us from the harmful effects of radiation and pollution.

Zinc is essential for the normal growth and development of reproductive organs and is required for normal prostate gland function. It protects the liver from chemical damage, promotes a healthy immune system, and assists in the healing of wounds. Symptoms of a deficiency include acne, fatigue, hair loss, cracking or peeling fingernails, recurring colds and flu, and slow healing of wounds.

If the thought of taking handfuls of minerals pills each day is a bit daunting, there are many ways to get your daily dose of minerals. One of the easiest methods is to simply drink them down in a liquid supplement. I recommend an all-natural concentrated Collodial Minerals containing more than 70 collodial minerals per serving made by Dr. Saxion's Silver Creek Labs (silvercreeklabs.com or call 800-493-1146).

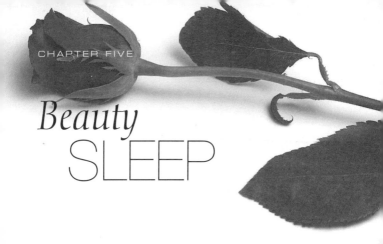

CHAPTER FIVE

Beauty SLEEP

O NE of the secrets of anti-aging and a healthy body is getting sufficient restful sleep. For most people that means between 7 and 8 hours of sleep on average. The reason it is so necessary is that as you sleep your skin makes twice as many new cells as during the waking hours. It has been shown that people who are sleep deprived end up with lower levels of a growth hormone the skin needs to repair environmental damage and tissue regeneration. But sleep is not only essential for vibrant skin, it is also essential to your overall health, muscle tone, and efficient fat-burning.

It has been estimated that from 40 to 70 million

Americans have chronic sleep-related problems, and stress and anxiety are the biggest culprits. Miss a few restful nights and we fall into a cycle of worrying about sleeping, which only aggravates the situation. And if you're tired, it decreases your concentration and memory, physical stamina, and emotional well-being.

TIPS FOR SLEEPING

- Commit yourself to the adequate amount of time for sleep.
- Regular morning or afternoon exercise is important to sleep, but do not exercise for four hours before bedtime. To exercise shortly before bedtime can impede your ability to fall asleep.
- Do not take naps or doze off watching television, even if you're tired. Your body functions best on a rhythmic schedule. This means going to bed and waking up at the same time, even on weekends.
- Keep your bedroom quiet, dark, and cool. If possible, use your bedroom only for sex and sleeping. Learn to associate your bedroom with sleep and not with computer work or television.
- Cut the caffeine, nicotine, and alcohol for at least 4 to 6 hours before bedtime. This means no coffee, colas, non-cola soft drinks, or chocolate.

Alcohol may seem to make you sleepy, but it increases the number of times you wake up.

- Warm baths raise your body temperature and ease tense muscles, but it is the drop in body temperature that brings on drowsiness.

- A bedtime snack increases serotonin to your brain to aid in sleep. Dairy products, bananas, peanut butter, and turkey contain tryptophan, a natural tranquilizer. Chamomile tea also works well. Avoid a late heavy meal, which sends your digestive system into overdrive.

- Many doctors suggest taking an herbal sleep aid such as melatonin.

- Develop your own sleep rituals. Try relaxation techniques, such as deep breathing exercises, and books on tape or tranquil music to lull you into dreamland.

- If you can't sleep after 20 to 30 minutes, get up and do something relaxing, such as reading, until you feel sleepy again. Don't lie there worrying about problems.

- For serious conditions such as sleep apnea and chronic insomnia, see your doctor.

Stress Reduction
and Your Own
VIRTUAL SPA

L IFE is full of physical and emotional and mental stresses. Your body is specially designed to allocate energy, oxygen, and blood to deal with these. The adrenal glands help the body adjust to sudden stress by releasing adrenaline, cortisol, and other hormones, preparing us for "fight or flight." For example, they increase the speed and strength of the heartbeat and raise the blood pressure and tense the muscles.

But stresses tend to overstimulate or whip the adrenals to produce cortisone. When this happens, vital calcium is pulled from the body's bones, sugar from the liver, and protein from the muscles. Over time, stress exhausts the entire body and takes a toll on your emotional well-being and overall health and natural beauty, which opens the door to new illnesses as well as aggravating existing health problems.

There is an ancient Chinese proverb that states: "Tension is who you think you should be. Relaxation is who you are." Janice Cox, lamasbeauty.com correspondent and author of three books on *Natural Beauty,* says, "This simple statement is so true. Learning to relax is all about learning to be yourself. We all live full, busy lives. Learning to unwind should be an important part of our everyday routine."

It is of utmost importance that you learn ways to de-stress yourself. Much has been written about this—a favorite hobby, journaling, reading, exercise, sex, meditation, enjoying your children, watching a funny movie, etc. But the best way to relax seems to be in the bath! "Nothing," Cox says, "is more indulgent or satisfying than to fill the tub with hot water, close the door, and soak. It is amazing how in 15 to 20 minutes all the 'have to dos' seem to fall into place and problems go down the drain with the bathwater."

Can't afford the time or expense of a week or even a day at your favorite spa? Don't fret. You can create a *spa-like atmosphere* right at home with a few basics products, tips, and your own ingenuity.

YOUR OWN VIRTUAL SPA

What makes a spa so wonderful is the sense of relaxation, tranquility, and peace it offers. Set aside an evening or afternoon when you'll be alone and create that setting right at home. While the sentiment of this virtual spa is directed to women readers, men should adjust to their own desires. All you need is:

- Soft relaxing music that you love to play in the background.
- Candles and incense placed around your bath.
- Your biggest and fluffiest towels in your favorite color.
- Gather together everything you need for a manicure—polish, swabs, files, cuticle scissors.
- A robe or body wrap. Plus a pair of flip-flops or slippers if you prefer not to be barefoot.
- A fridge stocked with your favorite spa foods—a crisp vegetable salad, tossed and ready to serve . . . fruit and cheese . . . chilled fruit or vegetable juices . . . peach ice tea . . . mineral water with slices of lemon or lime.
- Unplug the phone. Turn off the TV.

HAVE AN AGENDA

What would a half-day at your favorite spa include? It might look like the one below, modified to suit your personal preferences.

Step 1: Start with 30 to 45 minutes of easy stretches and meditation. Another time you might go outdoors for a nature walk and fresh air.

Step 2: Then go into the bathroom and wash your face thoroughly. Next, head off to the kitchen and boil a pot of hot water—throw some herbs in if you like—to "steam" your face and help open clogged pores. For best results, drape a towel over your head to create a tent-like effect, and lean over the hot water for 3 to 10 minutes (it's okay to take breaks if you need to!) to open up your pores. Follow with a gentle exfoliant cleanser or AHA-based cleanser to get your skin incredibly smooth and glowing.

Step 3: Follow your deep cleansing with an intensive mask treatment. Smooth on a mask for your special skin type and lie down for 15 minutes. Cool slices of cucumber on your lids will give your eyes a wonderful rest while your mask works.

Step 4: Rinse off the mask and draw a warm relaxing bath with bubbles or aromatic oils. Let yourself soak for a good 15 minutes or so. Try it with the bathroom lights out and just a candle or two with soft music in the background.

Step 5: Turn on the shower and give yourself a brisk one, washing your hair with your favorite shampoo and conditioner while you're at it, if you want. Take the time to exfoliate your whole body with a loofa and a fragrant "special" soap or bath gel followed by a grainy exfoliant to remove dead cells and soften rough areas.

Step 6: Towel off, and take several minutes to moisturize your whole body with your favorite body lotion or cream. Take the time to work it into those areas it's so easy to neglect, such as the soles of your feet and your elbows.

Step 7: Lie down again for a 20-minute deep relaxation session. Rub a little eucalyptus oil or your favorite fragrance in your pulse points to breathe in as you relax.

Step 8: Time permitting, let your hair air-dry if it's wet, to give it a break from hot hair dryers. If you must dry it, use the cool setting and gently rub your scalp with your fingertips to relax and stimulate it as you dry your hair.

Step 9: Bring out your manicure kit. Sit in a comfortable chair with something you can put your feet up on to give yourself a simple manicure and pedicure.

Even just adding polish to your fingers and toes will give you a sense of personal pampering and indulgence. While your fingers and toes are drying, close your eyes and meditate as you sit in your chair.

Step 10: When your nails are set, prepare your spa meal and eat it slowly, with pleasure. It's the perfect end to your virtual spa day!

CHAPTER SEVEN

Maintain a
YOUTHFUL
LOOK

A<small>T</small> some point you have to challenge the aging process or simply ignore the tell-tale signs. Unfortunately, many people surrender to the aging process . . . and look and feel like it. One secret of anti-aging I've learned from my clients is that there is a power—a real physical, mental, and spiritual power—that comes with how you feel about yourself. It comes out of feeling the best you can feel, and it affects how you care for yourself. So why not be your best at any age? You'll feel great and more confident, and when you feel your best, it affects your whole life positively.

BASIC SKIN AND LIP CARE

Keep your skin fresh, soft, and glowing! Nothing ages your face faster than the sun. Unprotected sun exposure will cause wrinkles around the eyes and mouth and ultimately can lead to skin cancer, but it will also cause lip wrinkle. I have written a whole book on *The Truth About Sun Exposure* that deals with this major anti-aging concern. Always wear lipstick or lip balm that contains sunscreen to keep your lips soft, wrinkle free, and young looking. Always protect your skin with sunscreen and never assume that a cloudy day or a pane of glass or being in the water is a safeguard against the ultraviolet rays—they are not! Use a foundation or moisturizer with sunscreen protection included. Be sure they have an SPF of at least 15. A sunscreen is so important these days given ozone deterioration. Ladies, never go to bed at night with your makeup on—your skin needs to be clean to breath and rejuvenate as you sleep.

Wear sunglasses that wrap around the sides of your eyes to help protect against crow's feet. Just be sure to purchase an updated pair of sunglasses that's suited to your face shape. There's no reason why at any age you should not be stylish with your eyewear. You can find an in-style pair of sunglasses at a drugstore or department store. And you can have prescription sun protective lenses put in the perfect frame for you. Don't be afraid to ask someone else their opinion when shopping for glasses.

NEW ANTI-AGING SKIN-CARE TECHNOLOGY

In years past, most skin-care products offered what I refer to as "hope and dreams in a jar"—big promises, but offering little in truly making a positive difference in skin's youthfulness. Recently, however, new skin-care technology has become available due to years of intense university studies and research. New products and ingredients are available that truly help reduce fine lines and wrinkles, the effects of scarring, and visible signs of aging, and help maintain healthy, youthful looking skin in general. Some examples of these ingredients are DMAE, Vitamin C Ester, alpha lipoic acid, Emblica, Argireline, and Matrixyl. My company, Lamas Beauty International, and a select handful of other beauty companies offer products that truly make a positive difference. I suggest you research products available in the marketplace that utilize these skin-care innovations and try them to see how they work for you.

MAKEUP

If you apply your makeup correctly, and if you stay current with styles, makeup will be your great ally in the anti-aging battle. The reverse can also be true if you don't apply your makeup correctly. I have written two books, *BeautyWalk* and *Beauty Basics*, that I guarantee will help you take the years off and capture your best look. I'll show you how to build the perfect look from the ground up, and how to make any facial flaws and creases disappear like magic. You'll discover the right tones that flatter your skin and eyes and hair at any age. It can make a 5- to 10-year difference in your look.

"If you're still using the same makeup and applications you used 10 or 20 years ago," says Diane Keelan, lamasbeauty.com contributing writer, "it's a dead giveaway you're aging. Toss that old stuff out and freshen up your look. Talk to an image consultant, makeup artist, or professional in the cosmetic field. Stop making the same mistakes time after time. You'll be surprised at some of the new and innovative products available in the cosmetic and skin-care world."

JUST THE RIGHT CLOTHING

Keelan adds, "Nothing can take years off your look faster than the right clothes. But changing the way you dress will push you outside your comfort zone, so you have to be open-minded and try new things. Have fun with it! If you don't try new things, experiment a little, you date yourself a little more each year!"

Just because you are aging, and your body is changing, does not mean you can't look great every day. Be aware of changes in styles of clothing and train your eye for what looks good on you. Make certain you keep finding a fit that gives you the best look. Toss out clothes that have gotten too tight—they make you look 10 to 20 pounds heavier. Keeping a youthful appearance does not mean being trendy, but it does mean current and updated.

"Why settle for clothing that makes you look or feel less than terrific?" asks Susan Kleinman, another contributing writer to lamasbeauty.com. "It really is possible—if you're willing to spend a bit more time shopping, and to wear a few great outfits frequently rather than stuffing your closet with near misses—to leave the house feeling like a million bucks every single day. Focus on clothes that make you feel fabulous and stylish. If you find a suit, skirt, or pair of slacks you love, buy it in several colors. No one will notice that the cut is identical—they'll be too busy wondering why you always look so good."

To be amazing on the outside as well as on the inside = true beauty.

CHAPTER EIGHT

Friendships, Love,
AND ROMANCE

STUDIES have shown that people who have a network of friends and family have lower rates of depression, infectious diseases, eating-related disorders, and body-image disorders. Other studies have shown that on the average, lonely people died younger, while healthy relationships extend our lives. People who are close to us help us get through tough times and make a significant difference in how quickly we age. Being created by God as social creatures, it makes sense that the health of our friendships and loving relationships will profoundly affect our health.

FRIENDSHIPS

Friends are a powerful factor in the battle against aging. In times of stress, which we know takes its toll on our health, friends are a boost to both our emotional and physical health. Gerald Ellison, Ph.D., director of Psychoneuroimmunology Services at Cancer Treatment Centers of America says, "Friends keep us from becoming isolated and lonely; they offer encouragement and support; and they help keep our thinking in line with the real world.... When we're missing friendship, we experience isolation and loneliness. These feelings are associated with illness, discomfort, and general ineffectiveness as a person.... Having friends can also be especially helpful if you're already seriously ill.... Friends—if supportive and encouraging—can increase our hope when dealing with illness and trauma. And increased hope is associated with higher levels of immune system functioning."

Do not let aging or busyness deplete your circle of friends. Seek out friends wherever you find yourself, and determine to keep adding new friends to your life. It's never too late to make friends, even best friends. Get out in the community and expand your circle of acquaintances. Involve yourself in organizations or clubs in which it is easy to make friends.

And don't allow life to cause you to lose contact with friends. If life stops you from interacting with friends, let them know why. Tell them you'll be back in touch after life settles down. If you don't tell them why you're not communicating, friends may start imagining the worst. Also, remember important dates such as your friend's birthday or Mother's Day. Send a card and make that call. Friends and loved ones are far too valuable to lose through a lack of communication.

LOVE AND ROMANCE

"Ah, love!" says Carol Ritberger, Ph.D., a lamas-beauty.com contributor and author of *What Color Is Your Personality?* "It can make our hearts sing or, figuratively, bring us to our knees. When love is present in our lives, the challenges of life seem less burdensome, and the perception we have of ourselves expands. We find that we no longer see ourselves as being separate from one another, but rather connected to one another. The world becomes a more peaceful place and our tolerance for the differences in people changes—it increases. Love is the gift of life, and our reward for reaching out and caring about others. Its magic transforms how we see things and encourages us to lighten up so that we can enjoy the delightful, tantalizing opportunities that come our way."

Love is the single strongest motivator of human behavior. Unfortunately, most of us don't place a high enough priority on our marriages and marital skills (as is reflected in our staggering divorce rates). Michael Brickey, Ph.D. and author of *Defy Aging*, noted that over the period of a couple decades, John Gottman carefully researched more than 2,000 couples. He found several principles that distinguish marriages that work. One principle is that successful couples know a lot about each other. Another principle is that they have mostly fond memories about their relationship. A third is their interactions have at least five times as many positive interactions as negative interactions.

Dr. Brickey adds, "Each of these is in your control. All you have to do to learn more about your spouse is ask. You can choose to recall fond memories and let negative ones wither or see the humor in them. You can make an effort to have more positive interactions and become aware of when you are starting a negative interaction."

The problem usually begins when we start to take each other for granted. While it's comforting to know you can depend on each other, the danger comes when dullness creeps in. If you feel your relationship falls into the "dull" category, it's time to spice it up again with some romance. When a relationship feels dull, sex suffers. And when sex suffers, so does the relationship. One easy way to put the zing back into sex and your relationship is to look for ways to improve your sexual skills. Dr. Bob Schwartz, author of *The One Hour Orgasm*, says, "A long-lasting, loving relationship is one of life's greatest rewards. Good sex only makes it sweeter. So why even think about spending the rest of your life without the best sex life possible?"

By the way, did you know that sex keeps you younger? According to medical experts, sexual activity releases endorphins, which lower stress. Regular lovemaking, which stimulates the hormonal glands, can also reduce the pain of arthritis and other illnesses. It is good for your heart, lungs, and skin. No other physical activity stimulates and refreshes so many systems of your body simultaneously as the arousal and gratification of sex. So get busy and start reaping the anti-aging rewards of frequent sex!

CHAPTER NINE

Lifelong Anti-Aging
SECRETS

WHEN it comes to anti-aging secrets, it is important that you form disease-resistant patterns of behavior that will be lifelong difference makers. In addition to the previous chapters, here are some of the things you can do:

THE POWER OF FAITH

Life can seem unbearable if you suppress emotions that are toxic to the mind and body, such as anger, hate, and guilt. It's tough when you're left to worry and fret about things you have no control over. On your own, it's hard to see life and its experiences from a positive perspective. It's hard to enjoy life and have a sense of humor when life seems meaningless and empty.

I cannot imagine going through life without the sense of peace and rest that my faith in God has brought to me. Our Father in heaven is both real and personal. As His children, He created us to love Him and to have a relationship with Him. Because He is here beside us, He knows our hearts . . . and our heart concerns. He knows our joys and our tears. We are not alone. He wants us to come to Him and place our worries and problems and guilt in His hands and to trust them to Him.

There was a time when I thought I could be satisfied with the things that the world had to offer me. It took a restless and unhappy heart to show me that God created me to never be complete or fulfilled until I possessed a living faith in Him. Faith is not a crutch for the weak. It is real and vital and always beautifies a person's life. To know that you are loved by God becomes the inner dynamic that will free you to be who you really are. It will empower you to always move forward and take new steps in your life no matter what you face. Don't try to go through life on your own.

THE POWER OF WATER

Considering that your body is 70 percent water, and

that even your bones are 10 percent water, you need a lifelong habit of drinking at least half your body weight in ounces of sparkling pure water every day. For every bodily function—from maintaining the balance within every cell to carrying nutrients to every part of the body to carrying the waste from your body—water is the key. Something as simple as a shortage of water can give you fatigue, stiff creaking joints, lung and urinary infections, headaches, dizziness, and constipation.

The health benefits from drinking plenty of water are enormous. Avoid drinks that dehydrate rather than sustain—alcohol and caffeine, such as coffee and soft drinks. Switch to herbal and fruit teas, and you'll be glad you did.

THE POWER OF OXYGEN

Oxygen is your greatest and first source of energy. It is the fuel required for the proper operation of all body systems. Only 10 percent of your energy comes from food and water, while 90 percent of your energy comes from oxygen. Oxygen gives your body the ability to rebuild itself. It detoxifies the blood and strengthens the immune system. Oxygen displaces and burns deadly free radicals, neutralizes environmental toxins, and destroys anaerobic (depleted of oxygen) bacteria, microbes, and viruses. It greatly enhances the body's absorption of vitamins, minerals, amino acids, proteins, and other important nutrients. Oxygen enhances brainpower and memory. Increased oxygen lowers the resting heart rate and strengthens the contraction of the cardiac muscle. And the list goes on and on, much like the benefits of water.

Maintaining proper oxygen levels in the body is a vital ingredient to health, vitality, physical stamina, and endurance. Healthy cells that have sufficient oxygen and nutrients manufacture enzyme coating around them that protects them from invasion. Yet you may be starving your body by simply breathing shallowly. It is reported that people in Western cultures barely use one-fifth of the lung's capacity to increase the oxygen flow to their bodies. The quickest way to increase oxygen levels is to daily practice deep-breathing techniques, exercise regularly, eat a healthy diet, and drink good clean water.

THE POWER OF DETOXIFICATION

One of the most basic steps you can take to give your body the chance to cleanse itself of impurities and renew itself from within is through detoxification.

The cumulative effect of our poor diet habits, lack of exercise, breathing in pollution and cigarette smoke, contact with harmful chemicals and pesticides, preservatives in our foods, and daily stress take their toll and overwhelm our system's ability to remove the toxins.

Detoxification is the cleansing process of toxins from your body that is going on inside you every second of your life. A detoxification program is for the purpose of aiding your body in these natural processes. Countless methods have been developed—from simply drinking more water to long-term fasting—and I recommend that you explore them. My good friend, Dr. Valerie Saxion, has written a small book, *How to Detoxify and Renew Your Body From Within*, that will guide you through the simple process of giving your body the opportunity to start feeling great again.

CONCLUSION

A century ago, people in their late forties were considered old. Today that same age group is wrestling with mid-life issues. Modern medicine has worked and is working to extend our life spans and has transformed our concept of aging. Anti-aging is a total life commitment that can help your years be youthful, vibrant, and healthy. Blessings to you as you make the daily changes to maintain your youth at any age!

> *"Beauty is in the eye of the beholder . . .*
> *but it is also in the eye of the possessor.*
> *What makes us truly attractive to others*
> *is the projection of our self-esteem."*
> —PETER LAMAS

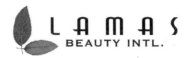

PETER LAMAS is Founder of Lamas Beauty International as well as its principal product developer. Lamas Beauty International is one of the fastest growing and respected natural beauty products manufacturers in the United States. Their award-winning products are regarded as among the cleanest, purest, and most innovative in the beauty industry—products that are a synergy of *Beauty, Nature, and Science*. The company philosophy is to produce products that are safe, effective, free of harmful chemicals, environmentally friendly, and cruelty free. They insure that their products are free of animal ingredients and animal byproducts.

All of the Lamas Beauty International products can been seen and ordered from their web site, www.lamasbeauty.com. To contact them for a complete product catalog and order form or to place an order, please call toll free (888) 738-7621, Fax (713) 869-3266, or write:

LAMAS BEAUTY INTERNATIONAL
5535 Memorial Drive Ste. #F355
Houston, TX 77007

Lamas Beauty offers a full range of hair-care, body-care, and skin-care products. Some of the most recommended products include the following:

Pro-Vita C Vital Infusion Complex: Highly potent anti-aging cream that helps improve premature aging skin. Applied nightly, it defends, nourishes, and stimulates skin through a combination of three powerful antioxidants—*Vitamin C-Ester*, *Alpha Lipoic Acid*, and *DMAE* —all of which fight free radicals and help restore firm, supple, youthful-looking skin. Advanced delivery system encourages the skin's ability to regenerate, increases the skin's firmness and elasticity, minimizes the appearance of fine lines and wrinkles, and helps nurture mature skin.

Pro-Vita C Moisturizer SPF 15: Distinguished as "Product of the Year" by *Health Magazine*, as judged by dermatologists across the United States. A potent, multi-action formula to maximize protection during the day. Contains a high percentage of highly absorbable L-Ascorbic Vitamin C (one of nature's most powerful antioxidants), SPF 15 sunscreen protection against ultraviolet rays (UVA, UVB, and UVC rays), Hyaluronic Acid for intensive moisturizing, Vitamins A and E and Retinyl Palmitate (a derivative of wrinkle-smoothing Retin-A) in a unique delivery system.

Chinese Herb Stimulating Shampoo: A therapeutic special-care formula empowered with Chinese herbs used for centuries to promote healthy hair growth, stimulate and energize weak hair and scalp. Gently removes hair follicle-blocking sebum and debris that can slow growth and cause premature hair loss. This formula is mild and gentle and won't irritate, strip away color, or dehydrate hair or scalp. Helps alleviate dandruff and itchiness.

Firming & Brightening Eye Complex: Distinguished as "Product of the Year" by *DaySpa Magazine*. The major benefit of this anti-aging eye cream is its ability to lighten dark shadows and circles under the eyes through the unique natural ingredient, *Emblica*, which is extracted from the *Phyllanthus Emblica fruit* (a medicinal plant used in Ayurvedic medicine). Emblica has been shown to soften age signs, deep wrinkles, and lines as much as 68–90 percent in independent tests. Also provides intensive moisturization through Hyaluronic Acid, one of the most effective and expensive moisturizing ingredients available.

Unleash Your Greatness

AT BRONZE BOW PUBLISHING WE ARE COMMITTED
to helping you achieve your **ultimate potential**
in functional athletic strength, fitness, natural
muscular development, and all-around superb
health and youthfulness.

Our books, videos, newsletters, Web sites, and training seminars will bring you the very latest in scientifically validated information that has been carefully extracted and compiled from leading scientific, medical, health, nutritional, and fitness journals worldwide.

Our goal is to empower you! To arm you with the best possible knowledge in all facets of strength and personal development so that you can make the right choices that are appropriate for *you*.

Now, as always, **the difference between greatness and mediocrity** begins with a choice. It is said that knowledge is power. But that statement is a half truth. Knowledge is power only when it has been tested, proven, and applied to your life. At that point knowledge becomes wisdom, and in wisdom there truly is *power*. The power to help you choose wisely.

So join us as we bring you the finest in health-building information and natural strength training strategies to help you reach your ultimate potential.

FOR INFORMATION ON ALL OUR EXCITING NEW SPORTS AND FITNESS PRODUCTS, CONTACT

BRONZE BOW PUBLISHING
2600 East 26th Street
Minneapolis, MN 55406

WEB SITES
www.bronzebowpublishing.com
www.masterlevelfitness.com

612.724.8200   Toll Free **866.724.8200**   FAX **612.724.899**